THE LITTLE BOOK OF
BEING

Vegan

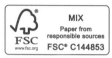

First published in 2021 by OH!
An Imprint of Welbeck Non-Fiction Limited,
part of Welbeck Publishing Group.
Based in London and Sydney.
www.welbeckpublishing.com

Disclaimer:
This book is intended for general informational purposes only and should not be relied upon as recommending or promoting any specific practice, diet or method of treatment. It is not intended to diagnose, advise, treat or prevent any illness or condition and is not a substitute for advice from a professional practitioner of the subject matter contained in this book. You should not use the information in this book as a substitute for medication, nutritional, diet, spiritual or other treatment that is prescribed by your practitioner. The publisher makes no representations or warranties with respect to the accuracy, completeness or currency of the contents of this work, and specifically disclaim, without limitation, any implied warranties of merchantability or fitness for a particular purpose and any injury, illness, damage, death, liability or loss incurred, directly or indirectly from the use or application of any of the contents of this book. Furthermore, the publisher is not affiliated with and does not sponsor or endorse any uses of or beliefs about in any way referred in this book.

ISBN 978-1-80069-010-3

Compiled by: Susan Clark
Editorial: Lisa Dyer
Project manager: Russell Porter
Design: Tony Seddon
Production: Freencky Portas

A CIP catalogue record for this book is available from the British Library

Printed in China

10 9 8 7 6 5 4 3 2

Illustrations: Freepik.com

THE LITTLE BOOK OF
BEING

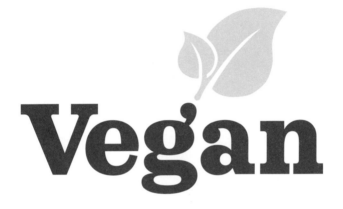

Vegan

A CELEBRATION OF
PLANT-BASED LIVING

CONTENTS

INTRODUCTION

In just a few years the idea of being a vegan has gone from a fringe dietary choice to mainstream status.

Whether you're no longer eating animal products to stop animal cruelty, to help save the planet, to look after your health or a combination of all those reasons, you are contributing to a more mindful, ethical and responsible way of living by considering the impact of your lifestyle and purchasing choices.

With the rise of people identifying as vegan has come a food industry scrambling to catch up. The days of a bland vegan diet of rice and beans — or getting stuck with fries and salad if eating out — are thankfully over because the race is on to invent more interesting and varied animal-free food. There's one company growing "clean meat" from animal cells in order to stop the slaughter of billions of farmed animals and another replicating Southern-fried chicken using plant ingredients.

Thanks to social media, there's no shame in telling people you want to put a stop to horrifically cruel practices just to put a steak on the plate and it's never been easier to eat well without eating anything derived from animals.

Veganism has permeated almost everything we buy, from beauty and health to fashion and home products. Being a vegan is not just about what you eat. It's about all your choices and trying to eliminate animal products from everything you buy and use; from your makeup brushes to your shoes.

If you're a newby interested in embarking on the animal-free journey, a part-time vegan or already a devoted vegan, you will find lots of information and inspiration on the following pages — including the effects of animal agriculture on the climate and the shocking practices involved, options for meat-free eating and the many health benefits.

In fact, in becoming vegan, you'll be keeping some pretty impressive company, from those who started the movement in the 1940s to the celebrity influencers switching to a vegan lifestyle today.

CHAPTER
ONE

The Planet & Environment

How your choices can help support wildlife, end animal exploitation, protect natural resources and halt climate change.

> **"**
> Never doubt that
> a small group of
> thoughtful, committed,
> citizens can change
> the world. Indeed, it is
> the only thing that
> ever has.
> **"**

Margaret Mead, cultural anthropologist

66

I've been a vegan for two
years... I'm motivating people
to do something about how we
are living on this planet.
We have to be about making
our planet more greener, the
urban areas more sustainable
for the children. We can't
just talk about it, we have to
be about it.

99

Stevie Wonder, talking in 2016

66

Opting for a sustainable vegan diet is the single most significant thing we can all do to help the planet.

99

The Ecologist website

An Oxford University
report showed that while
meat and dairy provide just
18 per cent of calories and
37 per cent of protein,
they use over **80 per cent**
of available farmland and
generate **60 per cent** of
agriculture's greenhouse
gas emissions.

A vegan diet is probably the single biggest way to reduce your impact on planet Earth, not just greenhouse gases, but global acidification, eutrophication, land use and water use… It is far bigger than cutting down on your flights or buying an electric car.

Joseph Poore, University of Oxford

Eutrophication: a big word describing a big problem.

This refers to the increase in phosphorus, nitrogen and other plant nutrients in bodies of water as a result of the run-off from farming, which results in less oxygenated water and more algae — thus a less hospitable environment for fish and a greater release of greenhouse gases.

The loss of wild areas to farming is responsible for the current mass extinction of wildlife. If everyone stopped eating meat and dairy, global farmland use could be cut by

two-thirds

– an area equivalent to the USA, China, European Union and Australia combined.

Where there's a will...

There are an estimated **570 million** farms across the globe, all of which would need to make slightly different changes to reduce their impact on climate change.

But with at least

$500 billion

paid out every year in farm subsidies, if the will is there to make those changes, there's a good chunk of money that could be diverted for the greater good.

Beef vs **Tofu**

Beef results in up to

230lb (105kg)

of greenhouse gases per 3½oz (100g) of protein, while tofu produces less than **8lb (3.5kg)**.

The Guardian

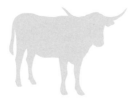

Beef vs **Peas**

Beef cattle raised on deforested land generates **12 times** more greenhouse gas emissions and uses **50 times** more land than those grazing rich natural pasture.

But even the very lowest impact method of raising beef is responsible for **6 times** more greenhouse gases and **36 times** more land than growing peas.

There are more vegans than ever before

The number of vegans increased by

600 per cent

in the
US from 2014 to 2017.

In the UK there were an estimated **3.5 million vegans** by 2018 — a huge increase from the 150,000 who identified as vegan about a decade previously.

Part-time veganism

In 2019, in the UK alone, a quarter of a million people pledged to go vegan as part of the Veganuary campaign run by the Vegan Society.

"

I'm a vegan. I respect
the environment
and I do my best to
spread the importance
of such an issue.

"

Jared Leto, actor and musician

66

We have a responsibility
to act now to minimize
our impact on this planet
— for our children and
future generations who
will inherit what we
leave behind.

99

Sir Paul McCartney, musician

An average-sized North American pig farm with 80,000 pigs needs nearly **75m gallons (340m litres)** of fresh water a year. A large one, which might have one million or more pigs, may need as much water as a city.

Equally, it takes nearly **220 gallons (1,000 litres)** of water to produce just **1 quart (1 litre)** of milk.

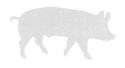

Water resources

Vegetarian author John Robbins calculates it takes **60lb (27kg)** of water to produce **1lb (450g)** of potatoes, but **20,000lb (over 9,000kg)** of water to produce **1lb (450g)** of beef.

Deforestation facts

🫘 For three decades now, global agribusiness has turned to tropical rainforests to grab land that can be used to either graze cattle or grow palm oil and soya.

🫘 Millions of hectares of rainforest have been felled for cattle to supply meat for burger chains and for animal feed farms to supply Europe, China and Japan.

🫘 Nearly 30 per cent of the available ice-free surface area of the planet is now used by livestock, or for growing food for those animals.

🫘 As soya becomes the world's major crop for chicken feed, so the food industry is driving cattle ranching deeper into the forests and, as a result, driving wildlife out.

🫘 Livestock now consumes the majority of the world's crops, while one billion people go hungry every day.

66

Do the best you can until you know better. Then when you know better, do better.

99

Maya Angelou, poet

Feed the world

Academics calculate that if the grain fed to animals in western countries were consumed directly by people instead, we could feed at least twice as many people — and possibly far more — than we do now.

It's just not sustainable!

A Bangladeshi family living off rice, beans, vegetables and fruit can live on an acre of land or less.

The average meat-eating American, who consumes around

270lb (122kg)

of meat a year, needs 20 times that amount of land.

Threat to biodiversity

According to the World Wide Fund for Nature — better known by the abbreviated WWF — one-third of the world's important 'eco-regions' are now under threat because of livestock farming.

More than half of the 40-odd global biodiversity hotspots, as identified by Conservation International, are now seriously and adversely affected by livestock production.

Poisoning the planet

Animal waste can be toxic to humans and wildlife. A cow excretes around **88lb (40kg)** of manure for every **2.2lb (1kg)** of edible beef!

Their manure and urine is funnelled into massive waste lagoons sometimes holding as much as 40m gallons (180m litres). These giant cesspools often leak or overflow, polluting underground water supplies and rivers with phosphorus and nitrates.

“

Only after I became active in women's issues did I realize that my veganism was related to those very issues... Dairy and eggs don't just come from cows and chickens, they come from female cows and female chickens. So, we're exploiting female bodies and abusing the magic of female animals to create eggs and milk.

”

Natalie Portman, actress

"

Becoming vegan is
the most important and
direct change we can
immediately make to
save the planet
and its species.

"

Chris Hedges,
Pulitzer prize-winning reporter

66

The problem is that humans have victimized animals to such a degree that they are not even considered victims. They are not even considered at all. They are nothing; they don't count; they don't matter. They are commodities like TV sets and cell phones. We have actually turned animals into inanimate objects — sandwiches and shoes.

99

Gary Yourofsky, animal rights activist

CHAPTER
TWO

Animal Welfare

With animal rights being
one of the main reasons for
becoming vegan,
here are some very real
facts behind the practices
involved in animal
agriculture.

66

There is no fundamental difference between man and animals in their ability to feel pleasure and pain, happiness and misery.

99

Charles Darwin, author of
On the Origin of Species

"

I chose to go vegan because I educated myself on factory farming and cruelty to animals, and I suddenly realized that what was on my plate were living things, with feelings. And I just couldn't disconnect myself from it any longer.

"

Ellen DeGeneres, actress and TV presenter

The message is out

With the rise of Netflix came the rise of advocacy documentaries that blew the lid off the secret world of the slaughterhouse and the cruelty that underpins dairy and egg production.

The basic message of the raft of films now available for public viewing is that animals are sentient creatures, deserve respect and should not be treated like commodities.

> **"**
> We don't need to
> eat anyone who
> would run, swim
> or fly away if he
> could.
> **"**

James Cromwell, actor and activist

66

Two out of three farm
animals are factory farmed,
meaning they are living
in small penned or caged
conditions and treated with
hormones and antibiotics
to prevent disease and
maximize their growth.

99

Compassion in World Farming report, 2015

We don't call pork pig — or beef cow.

Modern society has come up with many ways to help us detach from and disguise the real source of our meat products. Neatly packed, sanitized and drained from blood, supermarket meat bears little resemblance to the living, breathing animal it once was.

If you are in any doubt, take a visit to a butcher or slaughterhouse to see for yourself.

"

How can you eat anything with eyes?

"

W.K. Kellogg, founder of Kellogg's breakfast cereal

"

Could you look an
animal in the eyes
and say to it,
'My appetite is more
important than your
suffering'?

"

Moby, musician and vegan campaigner

According to the Vegetarian Society,
the average British carnivore eats over
11,000 animals in a lifetime:

1 goose

1 rabbit

4 cows

18 pigs

23 sheep and lambs

28 ducks

39 turkeys

1,158 chickens

3,593 shellfish

6,182 fish

The amount of meat* consumed in the UK is **175lb (79.3kg)** per year — which is **6⅔oz (217g)** per day, **4⅔oz (131g)** of which is red meat.

The number of UK citizens who maintain a vegetarian or vegan diet 100 per cent of the time holds steady at 2–3 per cent of the whole population.

*not inclusive of fish

Worldwide

80 billion animals

are slaughtered
each year for meat.

66

I know of no adjective
that adequately
describes the suffering
I have witnessed on the
factory farms
I've visited.

99

Deborah Giunta

As nations become richer, their meat and milk consumption increases.

Consumer demand for meat quadrupled in the last half century. In 2013, meat-eaters in Australia consumed around **255lb (116kg)** of meat per person, Americans around **243lb (110kg)** and Europeans almost **176lb (80kg)**.

However, change is happening and many high-income countries have started to see a stagnation in meat consumption.

Germany, Italy and France have all reported falls in meat consumption in 2020.

❝

Mother cows cry out for days after their babies are taken away from them. It's one of the saddest things I've ever seen in my life.

❞

Andrea Dowling

A voice for the animals

People for the Ethical Treatment of Animals (PETA) is the largest animal rights organization in the world with more than 6.5 million members and supporters.

PETA raises awareness of animal cruelty through public education, investigation, research, rescue, legislation, special events, celebrity involvement and protest campaigns.

Early animal rights

It could be argued that the animal rights movement started in India, given the widespread impact of both Jainism and Buddhism. Buddhists believe that all life forms, including that of non-human animals, are sacred and deserving of respect.

India still has the largest number and highest percentage of non-meat-eating vegetarians per head of the population of any country.

Anti-vivisection

The non-secular animal rights movement emerged in the 19th century with a focus on abolishing the abhorrent practice of vivisection — the use of live animals in testing for medicines and household products. Quakers, suffragists and humanists were among the most vocal of these groups.

Hunt campaigners

In the 1960s, the Hunt Saboteurs Association movement was formed in the UK to end hunting fox and other animals for pleasure. The organization then spread to Europe and North America

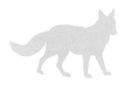

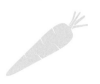

Animal liberation

By the 1970s, the argument about whether animals should have rights moved into academic and philosophic circles with writers and activists organizing in support of animal rights.

Australian Peter Singer was the author of the groundbreaking book *Animal Liberation: A New Ethics for Our Treatment of Animals*, published in 1975.

American Tom Regan published his seminal work, *The Case for Animal Rights*, in 1983.

66

What can you say about a society whose food production must be hidden from public view? In which the factory farms and slaughterhouses supplying much of our diet must be guarded like arsenals to prevent us from seeing what happens there?

99

George Monbiot, journalist and environmental activist

A champion of animals

Kind-hearted American Jean Clemens founded and worked with a number of societies set up to protect animals.

Jean — who sadly died in 1909 at the age of just 29 — was the youngest of three daughters born to Samuel Langhorne Clemens (author Mark Twain) and his wife, Olivia, who shared Jean's love of animals.

66

Thousands of people who say they love animals sit down once or twice a day to enjoy the flesh of creatures who have been utterly deprived of everything that could make their lives worth living and who endured the awful suffering and the terror of the abattoirs.

99

**Jane Goodall,
ethologist and animal advocate**

66

Our future selves will consider
meat eating to be barbaric.
I think we'll come to view [eating
meat] in the way we now look back
on the Roman games — having
crowds of enthusiastic people
cheering on the lions as they
slaughtered the Christians
or gladiators fighting each other
to the death.

99

Peter Singer, animal rights campaigner

66

I had never seen an animal die before. I had never looked my dinner in the eyes as its life drained away... And I will tell you it was a deeply unsettling experience.

99

Anthony Bourdain, the late celebrity chef

"

It was only a matter of time before the truth about animal agriculture was revealed. It's not in your face like racism or sexism — it's deeply ingrained in our culture, and financially ingrained, but now that it's revealed, people just don't want to be a part of that horrific industry.

"

Kip Andersen, filmmaker of *Cowspiracy* (2014)

"

A cow can live for 20 years, but dairy cows typically live to just their third lactation before being culled.

"

Compassion in World Farming report, 2015

66

Cows scream louder than carrots.

99

Alan Watts, author and speaker

"

It's a lifestyle, a
community, a culture,
an ever-expanding club
where the only price
of entry is being
mindful and making a
positive change.

"

**Motto of the Young Vegans pie and mash shop
in north London**

Main sources of animal suffering on factory farms:

1. Cages and overcrowding

2. Physical alterations like teeth-clipping or tail-docking

3. Unnatural light and poor ventilation

4. Inability to engage in natural behaviours

5. Breeding for fast growth or high yield that compromises health

6. Illnesses and injuries left unnoticed or untreated

American Society for the Prevention of Cruelty to Animals

CHAPTER THREE

Alternative Choices

Being vegan doesn't mean sacrificing good food or the pleasures of life. Here's why you'll never look back.

"

When I became vegan
years ago the alternatives
that were available left a lot
to be desired but now the
alternatives taste so good
that I can't imagine why
anyone would resist making
the change.

"

Midge Adler

A changing consumer

According to the Vegan Society, the demand for meat-free food grew by a staggering

987 per cent
from
2012 to 2017.

Vegan food is now being Googled three times more than gluten-free and vegetarian products.

Clean meat

Richard Branson and Bill Gates are just a few of the big-money names investing in environmentally friendly, slaughter-free "clean" meat.

Memphis Meats is developing a lab-grown meat from animals cells as an alternative to animal agriculture.

In 2018, the global vegan food market size was valued at **$12.69 billion**; a figure that is expected to increase by almost 10 per cent by 2025. Increasing consumer awareness about the benefits of following a vegan diet is cited as the biggest factor responsible for the growth.

A vegan lifestyle

Veganism is now used to describe a lifestyle — one that is against all mistreatment and exploitation of animals. In addition to food, the enlightened consumer wants their medicine, cosmetics and clothing to be free from animal additives.

Sales of meat-free foods
were valued at

£740 million

in the UK alone in 2018,
a rise from £539 million just
three years before.

Vegan fast food

Fast-food companies, from Greggs to McDonald's to Domino's to KFC have all launched vegan options. The trend for "dirty" or "junk" vegan also reflects the desire for more "comfort" vegan food.

Insta influencers

Social media has played its part in the rise of the plant-based lifestyle — from vegan recipes on TikTok to celebrities such as Ariana Grande and Miley Cyrus.

#vegan has more than 87 million posts listed on Instagram.

Veganism is a hot topic!

Just ask Google.

In 2009, the word "veganism" was ranked with a popularity score of just 33 out of 100 on Google.

A decade on, that popularity ranking has increased to 100 out of 100!

66

A human body in no way
resembles those that were born
for ravenousness; it hath
no hawk's bill, no sharp talon,
no roughness of teeth,
no such strength of stomach
or heat of digestion, as can be
sufficient to convert or alter
such heavy and fleshy fare.

99

Plutarch

Beyond meat

In August 2019, KFC trialled Beyond Meat vegan chicken nuggets at an Atlanta location and sold out in just five hours; selling the equivalent volume to a week's worth of regular popcorn chicken sales.

Top 10 best meat substitutes

1. Jackfruit

2. Tofu

3. Tempeh

4. Lentils

5. Seiten

6. Black beans

7. Veggie burgers

8. Chickpeas

9. Plant-based sausages

10. Plant-based chicken

GoodHousekeeping.com

"

We know we cannot be kind
to animals until we stop
exploiting them — exploiting
animals in the name of
science, exploiting animals in
the name of sport, exploiting
animals in the name of
fashion, and yes, exploiting
animals in the name of food.

"

César Chávez, civil rights activist

66

We can live as we were
meant to live — simply,
joyously, of and on the
Earth. We can live with
all our effort and with
pure happiness.

99

Scott Jurek, athlete and author

Vegan beauty

The vegan beauty products market was worth an estimated

$13 billion

worldwide in **2017** but the cosmetics market alone is set to reach over

$21 billion

by **2027**.

Don't forget your brushes!

Animal by-products such as hair and fur from a variety of animals such as weasels, squirrels, minks, badgers, ponies or goats are often found in makeup brushes.

For vegan brushes, look for those made from synthetic materials such as nylon and Taklon or a mix of the two. Nylon is a little more robust, so best for slightly firmer brushes while Taklon is good for a softer textured blush or powder brush.

"

Being vegan is a glorious adventure. It touches every aspect of my life — my relationships, how I relate to the world.

"

Victoria Moran, author of
Main Street Vegan

66

Not responding is a
response — we are
equally responsible for
what we don't do.

99

Jonathan Safran Foer, author of
Eating Animals

Know your labels

Not all vegan products are cruelty free, and not all cruelty-free products are vegan.

🫘 A product that carries a cruelty-free label (or rabbit logo) has not been tested on animals.

🫘 A product that is labelled vegan does not contain any animal products or derivatives but that does not automatically make it cruelty free.

Animal testing

Even when you buy a cruelty-free brand, you may still be buying from a parent company that tests some of its products on animals. If this is the case what should you do?

Some people think buying a cruelty-free brand owned by a company that is testing on animals just supports more animal testing. Others say any support of cruelty-free brands sends a strong message that the market is changing and the demand for animal-friendly alternatives growing.

You must make your own choice.

Vegan perfume

You may never know if your favourite scent contains animal ingredients because companies can list them simply as "fragrance", "perfume" or "parfum". But being aware of the following ingredients will help you to ensure your perfume is vegan.

Here's what to avoid:

🫘 Extracts of milk, honey, leather and beeswax.

🫘 East Asian musk deer and North American and European beavers are killed for their musk and castoreum respectively.

🫘 Civet, which comes from the anal glands of the endangered wildcat found in India and Africa, is often used as a fixative.

The civets are captured and held in cramped cages for years, with the musk "scraped" out every 10 days.

🫘 Ambergris, from sperm whale intestines, helps suspend perfume in the air. It is sometimes found washed up on beaches or floating as a rank-smelling fecal mass, but whales have been killed for it, too.

Sea sponges

Although some sellers of sea sponges claim to harvest only the top part of the sponge, which allows the animal to re-grow, a cloth or a plant substitute, such as *Luffa aegyptiaca* or sponge gourd, are much better options.

66

If you want to test cosmetics, why do it on some poor animal who hasn't done anything? They should use prisoners who have been convicted of murder or rape instead. So, rather than seeing if perfume irritates a bunny rabbit's eyes, they should throw it in Charles Manson's eyes and ask him if it hurts.

99

Ellen DeGeneres, actress and TV presenter

66

There will come a time
when the world will
look back to modern
vivisection in the name of
science, as they do now to
burning at the stake in the
name of religion.

99

Kathryn Bigelow, filmmaker

> **"**
> The greatness of a nation and its moral progress can be judged by the way its animals are treated.
> **"**

Mahatma Gandhi

CHAPTER
FOUR

Vegan Cooking

Here are food hacks and storecupboard staples to help get you started on your animal-free, plant-based diet.

"

Just how destructive does a culinary preference have to be before we decide to eat something else?
If contributing to the suffering of billions of animals that live miserable lives and (quite often) die in horrific ways isn't motivating, what would be? If being the number one contributor to the most serious threat facing the planet (global warming) isn't enough, what is?

"

Jonathan Safran Foer, author of
Eating Animals

Make vegetables the stars

Full of vitamins, minerals and fibre and available in an incredible choice of varieties, textures and flavours, vegetables take centre stage on the plate.

Experiment with roasting, stir-frying and grilling, and branch out with taste sensations, such as turmeric, cumin, chilli, five-spice, ginger and herbs you'd usually use on meat or fish, like rosemary or tarragon.

Bish, Bash, Bosh

Now known worldwide simply as the "Bosh Boys", when British digital marketing duo **Henry Firth** and **Ian Theasby** launched their first vegan cookbook it took the vegan world (and those just toying with switching) by storm, going straight to the top of the *Sunday Times* bestsellers list.

"It felt amazing to become vegan but we had to re-learn how to eat and how to cook... Everything we do has one intention and that intention is simple; put more plants on more plates."

Check vegan labels

Not all vegan products are healthy; in fact, many processed vegan foods contain saturated fats like palm oil and coconut oil and can be packed with calories. Cook with ingredients that are organic and as close to their natural source as possible.

Million Dollar Vegan

Take the Million Dollar Vegan pledge to try the vegan lifestyle for a month (31 days) and get all the help you need FOR FREE from this one-stop resource at: **www.milliondollarvegan.com**

If you need motivation, there are film and book recommendations and even inspiring speeches.

Once you sign up, you can access the starter kit, which includes meal plans, helpful nutritional facts and tips on eating out without missing out.

Debunking the myths
Myth #1 Vegan cuisine is tasteless.

Like any great cuisine, vegan cooking can be delicious; from raw vegetable sushi to barbecue tempeh; the possibilities will only be limited by your imagination.

Forget salads and rabbit food. Get creative with spices, flavourings and colours and get to know your plants, especially beans and grains.

Vegan food is only as boring as the vegan who cooked it.

Myth #2
Eating a vegan diet is expensive

Well, it can be, but it doesn't have to be; it depends on how and where you shop and, of course, what you buy. Follow these tips.

🫘 Although most supermarkets sell vegan ready-cooked meals, these are going to be expensive and never as tasty as making your own.

🫘 Stock your pantry with the essentials, switch canned beans for dried (which you may have to soak overnight).

🫘 Shop local and at farmer's markets for your veg power.

🫘 Don't confuse organic — which can be expensive — with meat-free or vegan.

🫘 Buy seasonal food that hasn't been flown halfway across the world. This is also a more environmentally friendly way to shop.

Myth #3 Vegans have to take supplements

Again, not necessarily true, although you do have to make sure you are not lacking in vitamin B12 and vitamin D3.

There are plenty of vegan sources for vitamin B12 including nori seaweed, Marmite and other yeast spreads, tempeh, fortified cereals and fortified milk alternatives such as soy or almond milk.

Sometimes known as the "sunshine vitamin", the body needs sunlight to make vitamin D3, but it is also present in mushrooms and tofu.

Storecupboard essentials

- beans (dried and canned)
- coconut milk
- coconut oil
- dried fruits and nuts
- grains including farro and freekeh
- herbs
- maple syrup (for sweetening and dressings)
- miso
- non-dairy milk
- nutritional yeast
- pumpkin puree
- spices
- tahini
- tempeh
- tofu
- tomatoes, canned whole and chopped
- vegetable and vegenaise (vegan mayonnaise)

Baking with flaxseed

Ground flaxseeds work well as a substitute for eggs in baking.

When you mix the ground flaxseed with water, the gum that is present in the seed coating becomes gelatinous, making it an excellent emulsifier.

The ratio for the mix is one tablespoon of finely ground flaxseeds to three tablespoons of water.

Use this quantity as the equivalent of one egg.

Tempeh vs **Tofu**

Tempeh and tofu are both processed soy products. Tofu, which is more widely used, is made from coagulated soy milk pressed into solid white blocks, while tempeh is chewy with a nutty, earthy taste.

Tofu is the more neutral of the two proteins and tends to absorb the flavours of the foods it's cooked with.

"

Peace begins with what you eat, wear, and use.

"

Gary L. Francione, author of
Animals as Persons

66

I don't see why
someone should lose
their life just so you can
have a snack.

99

Russell Brand, actor and comedian

Vegan kitchen hacks to change your life

🫘 Add black salt to your breakfast scrambled tofu for an egg-like taste.

🫘 Put a can of coconut cream in the fridge overnight. The next morning, whip with vanilla and powdered (icing) sugar to make whipped cream.

🫘 Use the liquid drained from a can of chickpeas to make a substitute for egg whites for baking. The liquid is known as aquafaba and will whip up with a mixer.

🫘 Warm up dairy-free milk before adding it to coffee to avoid curdling. Choose milks without fillers or added vitamins, which can leave an aftertaste.

🫘 Bananas, applesauce and nut butters make good and tasty alternatives to eggs.

🫘 Mash a can of chickpeas with ¼ cup of sunflower seeds or nuts and a little chopped onion. Mix with a vegan mayo to make a delicious tuna mayo substitute. Add dill, salt, pepper, hot sauce, chopped celery or grated carrots if desired.

🫘 Substitute avocado for butter in a 1:1 ratio next time you bake. It is really delicious in vegan chocolate pudding and cake recipes.

🫘 Nutritional yeast is packed with B vitamins and proteins — add it to sauces, popcorn, pasta and soups for a cheesy flavour.

🫘 Blend nutritional yeast with nuts, garlic powder and salt to make the perfect Parmesan substitute.

🫘 Soak cashew nuts in almost-boiling water for 15 minutes and then blend to make a vegan sour cream.

🫘 Missing bacon? Put liquid smoke on coconut chips, eggplant strips or tempeh for a much healthier version.

🫘 Run out of vegan mayo? No problem. Just blend soy milk, oil, vinegar and salt.

🫘 Add a tablespoon of apple cider vinegar or lemon juice to a cup of your favourite dairy-free milk, whisk, and let the mixture sit for about to 10 minutes to make buttermilk for baking.

"

I was not raised vegan. I did not become vegan because I did not like the taste of meat, dairy or eggs. I became vegan because, one day, I had the courage to take responsibility for my choices. I no longer believe animals are here for us for food, clothing, entertainment, testing or any other purpose. I am vegan.

"

Unknown

66

If you can't stand watching it being produced, you shouldn't be eating it.

99

Unknown

Good protein substitutes

Make sure your diet contains the protein your body needs to stay fit and well without meat; include seitan, tofu, lentils, chickpeas, many types of bean, spelt, spirulina, quinoa, oats, wild rice, seeds and nuts.

Some vegetables contain protein too, including spinach, asparagus, broccoli, artichokes, potatoes, peas, Brussels sprouts and sweet potatoes.

S is for seitan

"Wheat meat" has been around for centuries, although the name "seitan" (pronounced SAY-tan) is a much more recent development.
It is also called gluten, wheat protein or wheat gluten.

Made from wheat, seitan has little in common with flour or bread.
It is made by rinsing away the starch, leaving just the high-protein gluten behind. When cooked, it becomes very similar to the look and texture of meat, making it a popular choice for vegetarians and vegans.

Vegan cheese

Bland, pasty, chalky or just strangely uncheesy — vegan cheese can be a challenge until you find your favourite brand.

Happily, there are hundreds of variations — from smoked gouda to garlicky, herby cheesy spreads so don't give up. Start with these winners, which have picked up the best cheese awards.

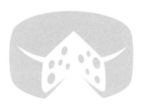

Violife Creamy Original Vegan Cheese was crowned the best plain vegan cheese in 2019 by cheese-lovers from around the world.

RIND'S Classic Cambleu is a soft-ripened, French-style vegan cheese, which recently scooped the gold award in the "Plant-based — other dairy" category at the 2020 Speciality Food Association's (SFA) awards.

Follow Your Heart Vegan Gourmet Cheddar is orange-hued and perfect for grilled or melting into a mac 'n cheese.

Vegan wine

Of course, most people would think that all wine — made from the natural process of encouraging grapes to ferment with yeast and produce alcohol — would be vegan. But animal products are used when winemakers want to "refine" the look or aesthetic of the wine.

Fining agents are used to remove molecules that are a natural by-product of the fermentation process but which can leave a wine looking cloudy or hazy.

For example, egg whites have been used to clear red wine, while a milk protein known as casein would be used to clear the haze from white wine.

Once the fining agents have done their job they are removed but they will, of course, leave traces behind.

As they aren't required to be listed on the label, you won't know if these are included. However, look for the words Unfined/Unfiltered on the wine bottle, which will tell you that animal products have not been used.

66

I am a firm believer in eating
a full plant-based, whole-food
diet that can expand your
life length and make you an
all-around happier person.
It is tricky dining out, but I just
stick to what I know — veggies,
fruit and salad — then
when I get home I'll have
something else.

99

Ariana Grande, singer

Vegan beer

As with winemaking, animal products are sometimes used in the production of beer to refine or clarify the brew.

The two most common animal derivatives used are gelatin and isinglass.

Gelatin is obtained by boiling skin, tendons, ligaments and/or animal bones with water; usually cows' or pigs'.

Isinglass is a kind of gelatin obtained from fish, especially sturgeon, and used for fining real ale.

You do not want these products in your beer!

"

Veganism is not about giving anything up or losing anything; it is about gaining the peace within yourself that comes from embracing nonviolence and refusing to participate in the exploitation of the vulnerable.

"

Gary L. Francione, author of
Animals as Persons

66

Always be the vegan
that you would've
wanted to meet before
you were vegan
yourself.

99

Vegan Twitter

CHAPTER
FIVE

Vegan Inspiration

Motivational quotes, fun facts and statistics to support your vegan lifestyle.

"

A philosophy and way
of living which seeks to
exclude — as far as is
possible and practicable —
all forms of exploitation
of, and cruelty to, animals
for food, clothing or any
other purpose.

"

Defining veganism, from the Vegan Society

The founding father

English animal rights activist **Donald Watson (1920–2005)** first coined the term "vegan" in 1944.

The founder of the Vegan Society, he used the new word to mean a non-dairy vegetarian. But by the following year, vegans were defining themselves as those who abstained from eggs, honey and animal milk, butter and cheese.

"

Veganism gives us all the
opportunity to say what we
'stand for' in life — the ideal
of healthy, humane living.
Add decades to your life,
with a clear conscience
as a bonus.

"

**Donald Watson, animal rights activist and
founder of the Vegan Society**

66

The vegan believes that
if we are to be true
emancipators of animals we
must renounce absolutely
our traditional and
conceited attitude that we
have the right to use them to
serve our needs.

99

Donald Watson, on the vegan philosophy

Veganuary

The now annual Veganuary campaign run by the Vegan Society in the UK was launched in 2014 to persuade non-vegans to try the vegan lifestyle for the month of January.

When it launched, **3,300 people** signed up; by 2018, this number increased to a staggering **168,000** with 84 per cent of those registered being female and 60 per cent aged under 35.

The perfect plant-based storm

While most vegans cite one or more of three key motivations for making the switch — animal welfare, environmental concerns and personal health — trend forecasters and market analysts say there's not one single cause for the rise in popularity of veganism but a perfect storm of factors, including the rise of social media channels and vegan cookbooks.

Plant-based is not the same as vegan

While the food industry may try to make the two words interchangeable, plant-based is not the same as vegan.

But using the term is a way to avoid using "vegan", which some people may still associate with sacrifice and a difficult-to-follow diet.

As the name suggests, a plant-based diet means filling your plate mainly with foods from plants, including veggies, wholegrains and nuts, while minimizing how much meat and dairy you eat. It does not mean avoiding all meat and dairy.

And while it may be going out under a new name, it is really a re-hash of the old "wholefoods" diet, which, similarly, did not eliminate meat or dairy.

❝

Whereas before, veganism may have been viewed like you were giving up something, now it's been reframed as what you gain.

❞

Kip Andersen, filmmaker of
Cowspiracy **(2014)**

> **“**
> If slaughterhouses had glass walls, the whole world would be vegetarian.
> **”**

Linda McCartney

66

I made the choice to be vegan because I will not eat (or wear, or use) anything that could have an emotional response to its death or captivity. I can well imagine what that must feel like for our non-human friends — the fear, the terror, the pain — and I will not cause such suffering to a fellow living being.

99

Rai Aren, author of *Secrets of the Sands*

66

The least I can do
is speak out
for those who
cannot speak for
themselves.

99

**Jane Goodall, ethologist and
animal advocate**

Unexpected V-gang members

Lizzo: Lizzo celebrated six months of veganism by posting a TikTok video saying: "As a new vegan, I'm enjoying exploring flavors from plants & plant-based proteins! Every journey is personal & deserves to be celebrated."

Thandiwe Newton: Inspired by her long-time vegan co-star Woody Harrelson, Thandiwe announced that she was going vegan in 2018 after the pair had starred together in *Solo: Star Wars*.

Sia: The Australian singing sensation switched to a vegan lifestyle in 2014 and subsequently joined the cast of the vegan documentary, *Dominion*, alongside Rooney Mara and Joaquin Quin. The film, released in 2018, exposed the dark underbelly of animal agriculture.

Venus Williams: The tennis superstar credits following a raw food vegan diet for helping her conquer an autoimmune disease, allowing her to stay on top of her game. She says: "Once I started, I fell in love with the concept of fuelling your body in the best way possible."

Benedict Cumberbatch: Voted PETA's "Most Beautiful Vegan" in 2018, the award-winning actor let it slip that he was vegan when asked he is had eaten anything "gross" to get in shape for *The Avengers* movie? He said: "No, no — well, I eat a plant-based diet."

Ellie Goulding: In January 2018, the singer announced her decision to go vegan. "Once I fully understood where meat came from ... I found that concept quite hard to live with. If you don't need meat to survive, I don't see why you have to have it," she said.

Jessica Chastain: the Golden Globe nominee went vegan after suffering low energy levels and says she has never looked back! "I just had more energy than I've ever had in my whole life. I was just listening to what my body was telling me!"

Jared Leto: The Oscar-winner and his 30 Seconds to Mars bandmates are all strict vegans. "Well, there was a time when we used to sacrifice goats," he says, "but then we all became vegans, so now we sacrifice tofu before the shows!"

Joaquin Phoenix: The actor was born to eco-conscious parents who raised their whole family as vegans. At the start of his career, Joaquin was offered several big commercial breaks in adverts for meat and milk products but turned them down. Now he's an ambassador for PETA.

Jennifer Lopez: "Jenny from the Block" went vegan to boost her flagging energy levels. "It's basically no dairy, no meat, everything is just plant-based and just from the ground. I love that I'm eating more greens. It makes you feel so much better," she says.

Tobey Maguire: The former Spider-Man shunned animal produce in favour of a vegan lifestyle in 2009. Tobey says the switch was easy because even as a child he struggled to eat meat.

Alicia Silverstone: Alicia says she has never looked or felt better than after turning vegan. "Once I went vegan, I lost the weight I wanted to lose, my nails were stronger, and my skin was glowing. I feel great and I look better now than I did 11 years ago," she says.

Still need a nudge?

Here are five films your fellow vegans say helped them to make the switch.

Cowspiracy — Crowdfunded in 2014 and later exec-produced by environmentalist, Leonardo DiCaprio, the film was dropped on Netflix in 2015. Prepare to be shocked. *What the Health* is the 2017 offering from the same filmmakers.

Okja — Sending a powerful if more subliminal message about animal cruelty, the film focuses on the friendship between a young girl and an adorable "super pig" by the name of Okja. One day their lives are torn apart when the animal is chosen to be the face of a new mass-farming initiative by the sinister Miranda corporation.

Food Inc. — Released back in 2008, but still powerful and alarming, filmmaker Robert Kenner explores how food consumption has changed over the past 50 years and how the meat industry has adopted more and more questionable (cruel) methods to supply the insatiable demand.

Supersize Me — The film is not about animal cruelty or animal rights, but you probably won't be ordering in a hamburger after you've watched it. Morgan Spurlock ate nothing but McDonald's for a month; gained 24lb (11kg) in weight, became depressed and suffered from sexual dysfunction.

The Game Changers — A celebration of the vegan lifestyle with contributions from Lewis Hamilton, Arnold Schwarzenegger and strongman Patrik Baboumian. The film, produced by vegan director James Cameron, focuses on former army trainer James Wilks, who spent months researching vegan diets after suffering a career-threatening injury.

Covert operators ...

When the actress Sandra Oh played Cristina Yang opposite Ellen Pompeo's Dr Meredith Grey, Sandra took the whole *Grey's Anatomy* cast out for a plant-based lunch at Truly Vegan in Hollywood.

Oh is known to invite friends to try a delicious vegan meal in the hope of inspiring them to make the switch. And clearly it worked with Ellen because the actress is now vegan, too.

A voice for animals

Singer, songwriter, actress and animal advocate Miley Cyrus adopted a gluten-free diet back in 2012 for health reasons and, two years later, switched to vegan.

In a tweet to PETA, she thanked the organization "for giving me the honor of receiving the Best Voice 4 Animals award! Living a completely vegan lifestyle, whether it's what I eat or wear, I am very certain that veganism is taking over and stoked to see so many brands jumpin' on this revolution!"

66

I'd rather bare skin than wear skin.

99

Pamela Anderson, animal activist,
actress and campaigner

It's a win-win for Pam

Baywatch star and former *Playboy* centrefold, actress Pamela Anderson, is another covert converter and voice for the animals.

She grew up in a household of hunters in Canada and turned vegetarian in response.

"I can't stay silent when animals are suffering or abused," she says.

Pamela won't even wear fake fur because she doesn't like the idea of looking as if she's wearing the real thing.

However, in a bid to stop Kim Kardashian and Melania Trump from wearing leather and fur, Pamela sent them both faux fur jackets.

And if that doesn't work, she's not afraid to push the other benefits of switching to a vegan lifestyle.

"Being vegan is an aphrodisiac diet. It's a win-win. Meat makes you impotent and unhealthy," she warns.

The eco warrior

While he has never publicly stated he is a vegan, Hollywood actor Leonardo DiCaprio — who won an Academy Award for his 2015 portrayal of a man nearly eaten by a grizzly bear in *The Revenant* — has invested in a plant-based vegan burger company called Beyond Meat.

The move was seen as the part of the actor's wider commitment to curbing climate change. When it comes to changing the world, actions count louder than words.

The fashionista

"I remember seeing a PETA ad and life as I knew it turned upside down. It was a video showing millions of pigs being buried alive. You could hear them scream in terror."

Canadian model Vikki Lenola has called out how animals are abused for the fashion industry and has taken an active part in protests. She led a PETA campaign against the use of coyote fur by Canada Goose — wearing nothing but body paint in freezing North American weather.

Meat is murder

The comedian Russell Brand hasn't eaten meat since he was 14, but he also gave up eating eggs and dairy more recently after watching the 2017 documentary *What the Health*.

In a video posted on Instagram, Russell explains that the Smiths' music influenced his decision to go vegetarian in his teens.

In 1985, the English rock band released the album *Meat Is Murder*. The album went to number one and the track by the same name influenced some fans — including Russell — to ditch meat.

66

You may choose to look the other way, but you can never say again that you didn't know.

99

William Wilberforce, slave trade abolitionist

CHAPTER
SIX

Mind & Body Benefits

If you needed any further convincing, here are the many wonderful reasons why a vegan diet is good for you.

You'll look better, feel great and live longer too!

"

Let food be thy medicine, and medicine be thy food.

"

Hippocrates

66

People eat meat
and think they will
become as strong
as an ox,
forgetting that the
ox eats grass.

99

Pino Caruso, actor

A healthier choice

Research shows that plant-based products help maintain blood pressure levels and lower the risk of heart disease, stroke, prostate cancer, colorectal cancer, cholesterol and premature death.

Generation gaps

Most vegans tend to be Millennials aged between 30 and 49.

Generally, younger generations are more environmentally aware and more likely to follow a plant-based diet than older generations.

Millennials are also more likely to say they've tried a vegan diet: **16 per cent** of Millennials have gone vegan at some point, along with **7 per cent** of Generation X and **8 per cent** of Baby Boomers.

According to UK Government statistics, one in five Millennials have now permanently changed their diet to reduce their impact on the planet.

Gen Zers are set to become even bigger consumers of vegan products. Research has shown that they consume **57 per cent** more tofu, **266 per cent** more avocados and an incredible **550 per cent** more plant-based milk than Gen Xers.

Kinder and healthier

While animal welfare remains the top reason that most people adopt a vegan diet, a Mintel survey of British adults reveals that half of those expressing an interest in making the switch cited better health as their primary reason.

"

All life deserves
respect, dignity
and compassion.
All life.

"

Anonymous

Look better, feel better

More energy, better skin, shinier hair and stronger nails are all reasons given for switching to the vegan lifestyle, but there are serious medical reasons for switching too...

According to researchers,
eliminating red meat from a
person's diet reduces
the **risk of death** by

12 per cent.

And people who follow plant-
based diets are **22 per cent**
less likely to have a heart
attack than people who still
eat meat.

A happier gut

The vegan diet increases the number of good bacteria in the digestive system as a result of higher consumption of fibre.

This then helps lower inflammation and so can improve both digestion and muscular aches and pains.

Less risk of diabetes

A plant-based diet, including vegan, will improve overall metabolism and help reduce the risk of Type 2 diabetes, which is linked to lifestyle choices.

You'll feel full for longer

With its rich variety of protein from pulses, such as chickpeas, lentils and beans, and high fibre, a vegan diet helps curb cravings for carbs and makes you feel full for longer, according to the *British Journal of Nutrition*.

You may lose weight

While simply becoming a vegan won't necessarily lead to dramatic weight loss, if you balance calorie intake against the calories you burn, then you won't want to reach for calorific snacks. Being more mindful about your food choices should make it easier to stick to your goals.

Helps heart health

A 2019 study has linked a higher intake of plant-based foods and lower intake of animal foods with a reduced risk of heart disease and death in adults.

This is largely due to the lack of animal fats which raise cholesterol, thus increasing the risk of heart disease and stroke.

Reduces arthritic pain

Because consuming animal-derived foods is linked to pain-causing inflammation, avoiding animal products can help alleviate joint pain, stiffness and swelling.

Probiotic plant-based foods such as fermented vegetables and non-dairy yogurts with live cultures can also boost the good bacteria in the gut.

"

Being vegan doesn't make you a stronger, better athlete. But it allows you to make yourself a stronger, better athlete.

"

Brendan Brazier, endurance athlete

66

I always say that eating
a plant-based diet is
the secret weapon
of enhanced athletic
performance.

99

Rich Roll, endurance athlete

Boosts energy

Studies have found being vegan can increase your energy levels. This is thought to be because your body doesn't have to use as much energy for digesting food — added sugars, saturated fats and carbohydrates all take your body longer to convert and slow you down.

You may live longer

A 2018 study in the
*Journal of the American Heart
Association* found that
a plant-based diet lowers
the risk of all causes of
mortality by

25 per cent.

66

If you think that being vegan is difficult, imagine being a factory farmed animal.

99

Davegan Raza

You'll feel better about yourself

Research shows that ditching meat and dairy is a significant mood booster and also increases mental clarity.

This is because the body can produce mood-enhancing hormones more quickly and more efficiently from vegan-powered fuel.

When people ask me why
I choose to live a vegan lifestyle, I
explain the ethical, environmental
and health-related reasons that make
me feel guilt-free.

Traditional western diets are the
leading cause of cruelty to animals
which occurs at the hands of the
meat, dairy and egg industries.

These industries slaughter billions
of land animals each year. Animals
feel pain and fear death just as
humans do. Animals on factory farms
live a life of mental,

emotional and physical torture
— they are separated from their
mothers at birth, confined to small
spaces, pumped full of hormones and
drugs, mutilated without any pain
relief, and violently slaughtered.

But choosing not to look at how
a hamburger, a glass of milk or an
egg is produced makes one just
as guilty as the people who are
slaughtering the animals.

"

**Deborah Kay Steinken, animal welfare
reporter and activist**

"

To get mud off
your hands, use
soap and water. To
get blood off your
hands, go vegan.

"

John Sakars, musician and activist

Follow the science

A study carried out by
Nobel Prize winner
Elizabeth Blackburn found
that a vegan diet caused more
than **500 genes** to change
in three months; turning on
genes that prevent disease and
turning off genes that cause
cancer, heart disease and
other illnesses.

And then there was ... a Global Pandemic!

Pandemics are an inevitable consequence of the poor hygiene, cross-contamination and low animal welfare that exists when we exploit animals for food.

Viruses emerge in live animal markets and in the filth and squalor of factory farms, and then can spread to people around the world.

To keep farmed animals alive in appalling conditions, they are given a potent cocktail of drugs including antibiotics.

Diseases become resistant to the overused drugs, superbugs emerge and we are left with nothing that can fight infections.

Our consumption of animal products drives this dual global health threat.

From *Million Dollar Vegan*

66

I can't think of anything better in the world to be but a vegan.

99

Alicia Silverstone, actress

66

Veganism is not a sacrifice. It is a joy.

99

Gary L. Francione, author of
Animals as Persons

"

The vegan diet is
healthy and leads to a
compassionate lifestyle.
I've gotten so many
benefits; my weight is
easily maintained, my skin
glows, I sleep better,
and I feel more energized.

"

**Meagan Duhamel, Canadian skater, holistic
nutritionist and Olympic gold medallist**